NF420496

Noni Fruit

The superfood that does it all!

By

Heinz Guenther Saenger

"Eat Your Food as your Medicine, Otherwise you will have to Eat Medicines as your Food"
– Dr. Michael Osae, GAEC.

owners, and this material is in no way affiliated with them.

Impressum:

No.4/2, Moo.7, A.Mueang, Ban Khok
67000 Phetchabun , Thailand
Tel.+66-96-480-4908 , hgs56@ymail.com

Table of Contents

Introduction

"Our food should be our medicine and our medicine should be our food."

–Hippocrates

The more we allow ourselves to be exposed to the natural world, the more there is for us to see. And people from all walks of life, from researchers to proprietors of specialized supermarkets, are continually discovering new plant foods, many of which have improved levels of beneficial compounds concentrated in their fruit juices. Noni has been consumed – and drunk – in the South Pacific for thousands of years. However, in recent years, it has been steadily finding its way into more health food staples, appearing in everything from beverages to dietary supplements[1].

The noni tree, scientifically known as Morinda citrifolia, has big, evergreen leaves and yellowish fruit. The Pacific Islands, Southeast Asia, Australia, and India are all home to this plant. The medicinal properties of noni have been extracted from the plant's roots, stems, bark, leaves, flowers, and fruit. In particular, fruit juice contains a significant amount of potassium. It also includes vitamin C, vitamin A, and a large number of other compounds, all of which have the potential to help activate the immune system and heal damaged cells in the body. Noni is also used for a variety of illnesses, including cancer, high blood pressure, dull sports performance, aging skin, diabetes, and many more; however, there is insufficient evidence from credible scientific studies to support these claims.

Traditional Tahitian healers think that the noni plant may be effective for a broad variety of ailments. According to the findings of a review of previously published human intervention trials, noni juice may provide some protection against DNA damage, increased blood lipid level, homocysteine elevation, and systemic inflammation caused by cigarette use. Human intervention studies suggest that drinking noni juice may also improve joint health, increase physical endurance, inhibit glycation of proteins, aid in weight management, help maintain bone health in women, help maintain normal blood pressure, and improve gum health[2].

In addition, the results of most of the research indicate that noni fruit has a much higher level of antioxidant activity than other fruit juices. The antioxidant impact of noni, as well as its interaction with the immune system and inflammatory pathways, may be responsible for many of the health advantages that have been seen in association with the consumption of noni fruit. The evidence that is currently available does, however, have some restrictions that prevent it from being applied universally to noni juice products. It is well recognized that different geographical conditions and differences in processing techniques may lead to the production of commercial noni products with distinct phytochemical and nutritional profiles. As a result, products derived from alternative sources of noni may have distinct toxicological and pharmacological characteristics.

This plant and its fruit are native to the regions of Southeast Asia and Polynesia where there are active lava flows. That's why its flavor is quite acrid, and the smell is distinct, earning it the nickname "stinky cheese" in certain circles. Noni has been used by the people of Polynesia as a component of their traditional and folk medicine for over 2,000 years[3].

Noni is most often taken nowadays as part of a juice cocktail. The juice has a wealth of powerful antioxidants and may have many other positive effects on one's health. This short book will explain all you need to know about noni fruit, including the nutrients it contains, the possible health advantages it gives, and whether or not it is safe to consume. So, Let's Get Started!

Chapter 1.
Introduction to Noni Plant (*Morinda citrifolia*)

When gaining knowledge of something for the first time, it's always best to begin at the very beginning! The noni plant is known by a variety of other names. In point of fact, even if you have never heard of "noni," you could have overheard one of its nicknames: Indian mulberry, canary wood, hog apple, or cheese fruit. Vomit fruit, because of its, shall we say, pungent odor; cheese fruit, as it's sometimes called in Hawaii, and we can only imagine that this is for a reason similar to the first. These are just a few of the less fortunate names that have been given to the noni fruit over the years.

Nevertheless, a simple seedling may be found hiding behind the facade of a worldwide plant of mystery. Growing in the aftermath of lava flows that is rich in phosphorous, the fruit has long been relied upon across Polynesia as a reliable source of food, despite the fact that it is not always desirable. In point of fact, noni is also occasionally referred to as a "starvation fruit," which describes its position in the hierarchy of fruit flavors. (In other words, native peoples would traditionally only consume the fruit during times of scarcity, when their options were something along the lines of "eat noni" or "starve to death.") And despite the fact that scientific investigation is in its infancy, there is accumulating evidence that noni might be something to make a big deal out of.

The noni tree is a small evergreen tree that may be found in the Pacific Islands, Southeast Asia, Australia, and India. Tubular in shape, the plant's white blossoms are pure white. The fruit has a surface that is pockmarked and yellowish-greenish-white in color. When the fruit is mature, it has a pungent odor that is reminiscent of cheese. In the distant past, noni was processed into a yellow or red dye for use in the textile industry. Additionally, it was used as a medicine for various diseases, and it was often administered to the skin [4].

Even in modern times, the noni fruit, leaves, blossoms, stems, bark, and roots are all employed in the medicinal process to treat a wide variety of conditions. However, there is no evidence to suggest that noni is efficacious when used in these ways. The Food and Drug Administration has issued many warnings to makers of noni products about the making of health claims that are not supported by reality.

Noni is taken orally for a variety of conditions, including colic, convulsions, cough, diabetes, painful urination, stimulating menstrual flow, fever, liver disease, constipation, vaginal discharge during pregnancy, malarial fever, and nausea. Noni has been shown to be traditionally effective in treating these conditions. Smallpox, edema, enlarged spleen, asthma, arthritis, other bone, and joint issues, cancer, cataracts, colds, depression, digestive difficulties, and stomach ulcers are some of the additional conditions that were treated with Noni in the past.

Patients suffering from conditions such as arthritis, high blood pressure, infections, renal diseases, premenstrual syndrome, migraine headaches, stroke, discomfort, drowsiness, diabetes, muscle aches and pains, menstrual difficulties, heart disease, AIDS, cancers, sprains, depression, senility, poor digestion, atherosclerosis, circulation problems, and drug addiction have been known to benefit from drinking its fruit juice.

The leaves have been used in traditional medicine to treat rheumatic pain and swelling of the joints, stomachache, and swelling brought on by an illness caused by a parasite known as filariasis. The bark was used in a concoction that was used to ease labor and delivery[5].

The noni extract is occasionally used to treat skin conditions. In addition to its role as a moisturizer, it helps fight the visible indications of aging. When treating arthritis, the leaves are wrapped around the joint that is afflicted. When treating headaches, the leaves are applied to the forehead. When treating burns, ulcers, and wounds, the paste of leaves is applied directly. A combination of the leaves and fruits is used to treat infections known as abscesses. Additionally, concoctions made from the root are used to treat wounds caused by stonefish and stingrays and as a salve for smallpox. People who have the leishmanial parasite on their skin might benefit from using an ointment made from noni stem.

Fruits, leaves, roots, seeds, and the bark of the plant may all be used for culinary purposes. There are several different chemicals in Noni, including potassium. It's possible that some of these compounds might stimulate the immune system, assist mend damaged cells in the body, and engage in a variety of other activities.

Other Names

Cheese Fruit, Ba Ji Tian, Canarywood, Bois Douleur, Hog Apple, Indian Mulberry, Jus de Noni, Luoling, Mengkudu, Menkoedoe, Mora de la India, Morinda, Morinda citrifolia, Mûre Indienne, Nhau, Noni, Nono, Nonu, Pau-Azeitona, Rotten Cheese Fruit, and Ruibarbo Caribe are some other names of Noni plant used in the different regions of the world.

Ethnic/Cultural Info

On their voyage across the Pacific Ocean to Hawaii, the Polynesians brought twenty-four different plants with them, including noni fruits. Because the bark of the noni tree could be used as a natural dye for fabrics and paper, the leaves, bark, and fruits were used in natural medicines, and the fruits were considered a famine food, providing nutrition in times of need, noni was selected as one of the vital plants. After the arrival of Polynesians in Hawaii, noni fruit trees were planted all over the islands, and they quickly became deeply ingrained in the religious, therapeutic, and cultural practices of the new inhabitants. The Polynesians held the belief that the noni fruit was a present from the gods. Pele, the goddess of volcanoes, is said to have a special connection to these fruits because they are one of the few types of trees that can survive in areas that have been devastated by lava flows and still produce fruit. In some Polynesian legends, the sour taste of noni juice is compared to the goddess, who is also described as having a fiery and sour personality[6].

Utilization in folk medicine and ethnobotany

Healers from Polynesia have used noni fruits for thousands of years to cure a wide range of ailments, including diabetes, high blood pressure, aches, pains, burns, arthritis, inflammation, tumors, the effects of age, and infections caused by parasites, viruses, and bacteria. In traditional medical texts from antiquity, the fruit is described as a key component of natural remedies. The flowers have been used to treat sore or irritated eyes, styes, conjunctivitis, ocular inflammation, and coughs. The fruit has been used to treat asthma, wounds, broken bones, mouth and throat infections, tuberculosis, worms, vomiting, eye ailments, depression, and seizures.

Historical uses of the noni plant

Ancient people living on the islands of the Austronesian archipelago made use of the plant as a source of dye. The bark of the multipurpose tree produced a pleasant reddish-purple mixture, and the roots of the plant, when boiled, produced a bright yellow color. Both colors have a significant place in Hawaiian and Indonesian cultural lore, where they were often used in the design of traditional clothing and decorative motifs.

In fact, the ability of noni to change color was believed to be of such great significance that it helped earn the fruit a prized spot aboard the canoes that ferried the island-hopping tribes throughout the South Pacific. This allowed noni to disseminate its seeds outside of the South Pacific.

Natives of Polynesia used to make a tonic and a paste out of the noni fruit to treat a variety of skin conditions, including redness, soreness, swelling, and other types of skin damage that can be caused by living in an environment with a lot of direct sunlight. Noni also has some traditional uses as a skincare product. In addition, new research has indicated that noni seems to have anti-inflammatory, antifungal, and antibacterial qualities, in addition to a plethora of antioxidants, all of which assist make it an appropriate ointment for the skin.

However, it is likely that the plant is concealing many more health advantages behind its putrid surface, which researchers are just starting to investigate.

Nutritional content

There are variations in the nutritional profile of noni juice. This is due to the fact that noni juice is sometimes combined with the juice of other fruits or given additional sweets in order to conceal its acrid flavor and putrid stench.

An earlier research that was conducted back in 2006 and published in the International Journal of Food Sciences and Nutrition investigated the various amounts of minerals present in over 177 different brands of noni juice. They discovered that several of the juices had varying quantities of a variety of minerals, some of which are listed below[7]:

- ☐ Iron
- ☐ Calcium
- ☐ Potassium
- ☐ Copper
- ☐ Magnesium
- ☐ Sodium
- ☐ Zinc
- ☐ Phosphorous
- ☐ Selenium

Because of these fluctuating ratios, it might be difficult to provide accurate nutritional information for any particular batch of noni juice. Noni contains a variety of phytochemicals and antioxidants, including the following:

- ☐ Flavonoids
- ☐ Lignans
- ☐ Iridoids
- ☐ Anthraquinones
- ☐ Coumarins

□ Terpenoids

□ Sterols

□ Fatty acids

□ Polysaccharides

Tahitian Noni Juice is the most popular brand currently available and is often used in research. It is made up of 11% grape and blueberry juice concentrates in addition to 89% noni fruit. The following three nutrients may be found in 3.5 ounces (100 milliliters) of Tahitian Noni Juice:

□ **Calories:** 47 calories

□ **Carbs:** 11 grams

□ **Protein:** less than 1 gram

□ **Fat:** less than 1 gram

□ **Sugar:** 8 grams

□ **Vitamin C:** 33% of the Reference Daily Intake (RDI)

□ **Biotin:** 17% of the RDI

□ **Folate:** 6% of the RDI

□ **Magnesium:** 4% of the RDI

□ **Potassium:** 3% of the RDI

□ **Calcium:** 3% of the RDI

□ **Vitamin E:** 3% of the RDI

Like most fruit juice, Noni juice includes primarily carbohydrates. It has high vitamin C content, which is critical for maintaining healthy skin as well as the immune system. In addition to this, it is an excellent source of biotin and folate, which are both B vitamins that play many key functions in your body, one of which is assisting in the transformation of food into energy. The nutritional makeup of noni juice might differ from one region to another.

Anti-oxidants

The significant quantities of antioxidants that may be found in noni juice are well-known fact. Antioxidants are substances that protect cells from being damaged by chemicals known as free radicals. In order to preserve its health to its full potential, your body has to maintain an appropriate ratio of antioxidants to free radicals.

Researchers believe that the high antioxidant qualities of noni juice are likely to be responsible for any possible health advantages of drinking noni juice. Beta carotene, iridoids, vitamins C and E, and other compounds are the primary antioxidants found in noni juice. Iridoids, in particular, have been shown to have a significant amount of antioxidant activity in test-tube tests; however, further study on their effects on humans is still required.

Despite this, research suggests that consuming a diet high in antioxidants, such as those that may be found in noni juice, may reduce the likelihood that a person would develop chronic diseases such as heart disease or diabetes.

Useful Alkaloids

The noni fruit has a significant amount of various vitamins, minerals, enzymes, and health-promoting alkaloids. It possesses xeronine, which is a very important alkaloid. Xeronine is present in the cells of all living things, including microorganisms, plants, animals, and humans. This alkaloid is essential to the proper functioning of every cell in the body and makes it possible for proteins to carry out all of the roles that are specifically assigned to them.

Because xeronine works with endorphins to alleviate pain and cause a sense of euphoria, it is the body's most powerful painkiller and a sedative that is quite effective. Even though a large number of people get xeronine from the food they eat, some scientists are concerned that this may not be enough. Because of the state of the soil and the health of the crops, many of the nutrients that we get from our food are being lost, and a deficiency in this essential alkaloid can lead to illness. In addition to xeronine, this plant also has proxeronine, which is an even more beneficial alkaloid. Proxeronine is the first step in the production of xeronine, and it enables the body to regulate the amount of xeronine that is produced, with the excess going to waste. This enables the proteins in the body to carry out the functions for which they were originally intended. Various essential amino acids can be found in the roots and leaves of the noni plant.

In addition, the roots of the noni plant contain a chemical known as damnacanthal. According to research, damnacanthal can successfully transform cancer cells into normal cells. The University of Hawaii conducted a clinical study with the goals of learning more about the usage of noni as a cancer treatment and identifying the compounds in the noni fruit that is responsible for its anti-cancer effects. In this study with mice with cancer, the use of noni extract resulted in longer survival times for the animals.

Chapter 2.

The Possible Healthful Effects of Noni Fruit

There are a variety of possible advantages of drinking noni juice. However, it is essential to bear in mind that research on this fruit is of a very recent period, and more studies are required to determine the extent to which many of these health benefits apply.

Counter the carcinogenic effects of cigarette smoking

There is some evidence that drinking noni juice may protect cells from harm, especially that caused by cigarette smoke. The inhalation of tobacco smoke results in the production of potentially harmful levels of free radicals. Excessive levels might lead to oxidative stress as well as harm to the cells. Oxidative stress has been linked to a wide variety of diseases, most notably cancer, diabetes, and cardiovascular disease. According to a number of studies, eating foods that are high in antioxidants may help lower oxidative stress.

Heavy smokers were given a daily dose of noni juice equal to 4 ounces (118 milliliters) in one research trial. After one month, they observed a thirty percent decrease in the levels of two common free radicals in comparison to their initial levels. Smoke from tobacco products has also been linked to cancer. Certain chemicals in tobacco smoke have the potential to connect to cells in your body, which might eventually result in the development of a tumor. However, noni juice does not undo all of the harmful consequences that smoking has on a person's health, and hence it should not be seen as an alternative for quitting smoking[8].

Improves heart's health

There is some evidence that drinking noni juice may improve cardiovascular health by decreasing cholesterol levels and reducing inflammation. There are a number of essential roles that cholesterol plays in the body; nevertheless, high levels of specific forms of cholesterol and chronic inflammation both have been linked to an increased risk of cardiovascular disease.

According to the findings of one research, consuming up to 6.4 ounces (188 ml) of noni juice on a daily basis for a period of one month dramatically lowered total cholesterol, LDL (bad) cholesterol levels, and the levels of the inflammatory blood marker C-reactive protein. However, given that the participants who participated in the research were heavy smokers, it is not possible to apply the findings to all individuals. Researchers are of the opinion that the antioxidants included in noni juice may help lower the elevated cholesterol levels brought on by smoking cigarettes.

In a separate experiment lasting 30 days, non-smokers were given 59 milliliters (about 2 ounces) of noni juice twice every day. Participants did not observe substantial increases in cholesterol levels. Based on these findings, it seems that both smokers and non-smokers may both benefit from the cholesterol-lowering effects of noni juice. Having stated that, there is a need for more study on noni juice and cholesterol.

Increases endurance during exercise

Noni juice may increase physical endurance. The preliminary findings of certain studies show that long-distance runners who consume noni, grapefruit, and blackberry juices over a period of 21 days might see an increase in their exercise endurance. In fact, people who lived in the Pacific Islands thought that eating noni fruit would strengthen the body so that it could better endure lengthy journeys at sea. Drinking noni juice before or during exercise has been shown in a few trials to have beneficial benefits.

For instance, participants in research that lasted for three weeks were given either 3.4 ounces (100 milliliters) of noni juice or a placebo twice daily. A 21% increase in average duration before experiencing exhaustion was seen in the group that drank noni juice, which is suggestive of better endurance.

Other human and animal studies indicate results that are comparable regarding the effectiveness of noni juice in warding off weariness and boosting endurance. It is possible that the improvement in physical endurance that is linked with noni juice is due to the antioxidants that it contains. These antioxidants may decrease the damage to muscle tissue that would typically occur during exercise.

Helps in treating arthritis

Because of its ability to alleviate pain, noni fruit has been used in the practice of traditional folk medicine for over two thousand years. There is currently evidence from studies to support this advantage. People who suffered from degenerative arthritis of the spine, for instance, participated in a trial that lasted for one month and were given 0.5 ounces (15 ml) of noni juice twice a day. The noni juice group reported a considerably reduced level of discomfort, with sixty percent of patients experiencing total alleviation from their neck pain.

People who suffered from osteoarthritis participated in another trial in which they were given 89 milliliters or three ounces of noni juice on a daily basis. After the first three months of treatment, they reported a considerable reduction in the frequency and intensity of arthritic pain, as well as an improvement in their overall quality of life.

The discomfort caused by arthritis is often linked to increased inflammation as well as oxidative stress. Because of this, noni juice may be able to give natural pain relief by lowering inflammatory levels and scavenging free radicals.

Boosts immune system

The immune system may benefit from drinking noni juice. It has a high vitamin C content, similar to that of other fruit juices. As an example, 3.5 ounces (100 milliliters) of Tahitian Noni Juice contains about 33% of the recommended daily intake for this vitamin. Vitamin C helps your immune system by shielding your cells from the damage caused by free radicals and other harmful elements in the environment.

Noni juice contains a variety of additional antioxidants, including beta carotene, which may also contribute to an improved immune system.

One preliminary investigation that lasted for eight weeks indicated that healthy individuals who consumed 11 ounces (330 milliliters) of noni juice on a daily basis had higher levels of immune cell activation and lower levels of oxidative stress[9].

Fights cancer

Initial investigations point to the possibility that ingesting 6-8 grams of noni every day might help persons with advanced cancer enhance their physical function and reduce feelings of weariness and discomfort. However, it does not seem that noni can lessen the growth of the tumor.

Stops spinal degeneration

Spinal degeneration due to advancing age (cervical spondylosis) may also be halted with the noni fruit. In comparison to physiotherapy on its own, a preliminary study reveals that consuming noni juice in conjunction with engaging in physiotherapy for a period of four weeks may decrease neck discomfort and increase neck flexibility. On the other hand, it seems that treatment with physiotherapy alone may relieve pain and increase flexibility more effectively than noni juice alone does.

Lowers hypertension (high blood pressure)

Initial studies show that those who have high blood pressure and consume 4 ounces of noni juice every day for a period of one month may have a reduction in their blood pressure.

Cures skin illness

A skin illness caused by the presence of parasites (leishmaniasis) may also be treated using noni. Early study indicates that putting an ointment on the skin that includes noni stem could alleviate some of the cutaneous symptoms of leishmaniasis.

Noni juice is also well recognized for the antioxidants it contains, and it also contributes to the skin's natural moisture balance. You may try applying the juice straight to your skin to observe how it heals and nourishes your dry, damaged skin. Therefore, if you have dry skin and often encounter patches on your skin, you may keep your skin moisturized by applying this juice to your skin and drinking it. Both of these methods will work.

Alleviates nausea

The noni fruit may help alleviate nausea. There is evidence that it helps minimize nausea after surgical procedures. On the other hand, it does not seem to have any effect on vomiting.

Aids in the treatment of fever and sour throat

Because noni juice has antiviral qualities, it is useful in the treatment of fever and sour throat. You just need to consume a small amount of noni juice in order to experience its benefits. It is important that you do not consume too much of it all at once.

Prevents aging

Most of us want to avoid wrinkles on our skin and have our skin become lax as we grow older. You may nevertheless slow down the process, despite the fact that it is a normal occurrence, by drinking juice made from noni fruit. Vitamin C and selenium are both abundant in the juice, and these two nutrients work together to combat the effects of free radicals, maintain the skin's suppleness, and slow down the aging process. People who are becoming older yet wish to maintain the appearance of being younger are encouraged to use it.

Encourages a healthy metabolic system

Although they are low in calories, noni fruits contain a wealth of phytonutrients, which are plant-based chemicals that exhibit remarkable antioxidant properties. In addition to eliminating harmful free radicals and protecting healthy cells from oxidation and damage, these help maintain optimal metabolism by converting food into energy for various biochemical reactions in the body. These reactions take place inside the body. Eating a small portion of noni fruits or drinking the juice prior raises levels of energy, protects muscle cells from wear and tear and improves exercise performance[10].

Beneficial for both the hair and the skin

Noni juice is the ultimate organic solution for rejuvenating skin texture and enhancing hair growth because it contains vitamin C, biotin or vitamin B7, trace minerals of zinc, copper, selenium, and phytonutrients. These valuable nutrients, along with a host of antioxidant and antimicrobial elements in the juice of the noni fruit, detoxify the body from the inside out, flush out toxins, boost collagen synthesis to turn back the hands of the biological clock, heal acne scars, and immensely enrich skin complexion. When applied topically, the antimicrobial properties in noni juice and fruit powder derivates soothe irritation, itching, dandruff, and flaking to supply a clean scalp and strong, thick, silky hair.

Treats certain other conditions

- Asthma
- Colds
- Colic
- Constipation
- Cough
- Depression
- Diabetes
- Digestion issues
- Enlarged spleen
- Eye cataracts
- Problems with the heart

- Infections
- Kidney problems
- Liver issues
- Menstrual difficulties
- Migraine
- Pain
- Slowing down the appearance of aging
- Seizures
- Smallpox
- Stomach ulcers
- Swelling
- Stroke
- Issues with the urinary tract
- Vaginal discharge

Consuming noni juice may have various beneficial effects, such as increasing your stamina, easing discomfort, bolstering your immune system, protecting your cells from the harm caused by cigarette smoke, and helping smokers maintain good heart health.

Chapter 3.

How to Consume Noni

It is quite difficult to get fresh noni fruit in the United States, but it is a common component in the cuisines of many countries in the Pacific, which is where it naturally grows. You'll never forget your first smell of noni, and its astringent fragrance is a good indicator of the unique taste it imparts. The acrid taste of noni, which is also known as the cheese fruit, earned the fruit its ripe name because it is comparable to the pungent flavor of Limburger cheese.

Do not allow the fruit's notoriously pungent smell to deter you from savoring the one-of-a-kind taste it has to offer. The flavor of ripe noni is quite similar to its aroma; it is earthy and compost-like, with a tinge of lemony sourness. It is common for the taste of ripening noni to be more astringent and intense in proportion to the hardness of the flesh. When it has reached its complete maturity, the flesh of the stinky-sour cheese reaches an almost gooey consistency, and the taste and aroma of the cheese are at their pinnacle.

The noni fruit starts off tough, lumpy, and green, but as it ripens, it transforms into a creamy yellow, then white fruit with smooth, transparent skin that looks like an oval-shaped potato. The inside of noni fruits consists of white flesh with plenty of black seeds that may be consumed. Some noni lovers opt to swallow them, despite the fact that their consistency is similar to that of wood. Raw noni may now be enjoyed as an exciting snack for those who are up for the challenge[11].

Before ripening, noni has a taste that is quite bitter and a texture that is exceedingly rough; it is only when it is cooked that it may be consumed. The use of noni at this stage imparts a taste that is bitter, fragrant, and earthy into rice dishes, curries, and soups. Even though noni has a flavor that may be unfamiliar to fruit lovers at first, the intricacy of its taste makes it well worth the effort to learn to appreciate it.

The method that you use to make your noni will be determined by the recipe that you choose. The following are the most frequent methods that may be used to consume.

Taking slices of noni

The noni fruit may be sliced differently depending on whether it is ripe or unripe. Prior to ingestion, the fruit must first have the rough peel removed while it is still in its green state, and then the flesh must be cooked. After removing the peel, the thick flesh of the fruit may be sliced, diced, or chopped in the same manner as the flesh of a potato or a carrot.

When noni has reached full maturity, the flesh within may be readily separated by pulling it apart with your fingertips. Noni may be sliced either by cutting it lengthwise into wedges or by cutting it across the width into circular slices.

Cooking Noni

Raw noni can only be consumed after it has reached its peak ripeness. Before boiling the unripe flesh of the fruit, it is best to remove and discard the green peel, which is particularly tough.

When it has reached its full maturity, noni has the appearance of a smooth, lumpy potato. Its flesh is transparent white and gives gently to the touch. As an exciting and novel fruit snack, try eating raw slices of fresh noni, complete with the fruit's skin and seeds. Don't forget to finish it off with a little sprinkle of sea salt!

There are numerous methods to counteract the intense taste of mature noni fruit. To give you an example, combine the fruit with a substantial cheese, starchy vegetable dish, rich sauce, or sweet rice.

Drinking Noni

Noni is often used in the cuisine of many different civilizations and is even considered an emergency food supply in certain nations. Juice made from whole fruits, either unfermented or fermented, is one of the most common methods for people to consume noni. The most frequent way to consume noni is in the form of juice, which may range in concentration from 10 to 100 percent. Particularly when fermented into a powerful, sour juice, noni is said to offer anti-inflammatory qualities in addition to other beneficial characteristics for the body. After being pureed and filtered, ripe noni may be processed into a fresh juice that is more complexly aromatic, with a hint of lemony flavor and an impact that numbs the lips.

The best method to get juice that is 100 percent noni is to make it at home. Just put the noni fruit in a glass jar after it has reached its maximum ripeness and add a very trace quantity of water. After that, make sure it is well sealed, and let the contents anywhere from one week to three months to organically break down and ferment in the container. At last, pass the juice through a cheesecloth strainer, and then put it in the refrigerator to chill. Note that noni juice is often combined with other juices in order to improve its flavor since noni fruit itself is not known for having the greatest flavor[12].

Storing Noni

Because noni fruits develop so rapidly and have a very limited shelf life, appropriate storage is essential if you want to make the most of these elusive delicacies. Noni that has not yet reached its full maturity can be kept for up to three days in a location that is cool, dark, and has enough ventilation. When a noni fruit is mature, it will change a transparent white color and become considerably softer. These ripened nonis should be consumed right away, or else they should be preserved in a glass jar that has a tight seal so they may be fermented.

When you first these strange fruits, you should consume them right away. If you have any leftovers, you may put them in a container that seals well and place them in the refrigerator for one day, or you can freeze the pieces. It is simple to freeze noni fruit after it has reached maturity. Wrap the noni fruit in plastic wrap and store it in a container that can withstand freezing for up to three months.

Chapter 4.

Consuming Noni Juice for Weight Loss

You may be wondering what makes this Noni juice so unique and how exactly it might assist you in your efforts to reduce body fat. Because it contains a high concentration of antioxidants and a diverse array of other nutrients—including vitamin C, provitamin A, protein, amino acids, and many others—that are known to treat a wide variety of illnesses, it has a long history of use as a weight-related medicinal remedy in some of the cultures that make up Southeast Asia.

In 2016, the World Health Organization found that 39 percent of people aged 18 and over (39 percent of males and 40 percent of women) were overweight. In all, around 13% of the adult population of the world, which amounts to millions of individuals, is overweight. Over the last many years, obesity has evolved into a major health risk for everyone. People often gain extra weight because they consume an excessive amount of calories, are inactive physically, and do not get enough nutrients in their diet. This causes a slowdown in their metabolism, which in turn leads to obesity.

Studies have shown that the noni plant has roughly 160 different phytochemical substances inside its tissues. The phenolic acids, organic acids, and alkaloids contained in the plant make up its important micronutrients. The principal organic acids are capric and caproic acid, while the primary alkaloid is xeronine. The noni fruit contains a variety of soluble solids, dietary fibers, and proteins in addition to its 90% water content. Protein and important amino acids including aspartic acid, glutamic acid, and isoleucine are found in relatively high quantities in this fruit.

There is a trace quantity of selenium in the noni juice. The noni fruit contains both vitamin C, often known as ascorbic acid, and the precursor to vitamin A, which is called provitamin A. Protein, glucose, fructose, potassium, salt, magnesium, calcium, and vitamins A and C are among the components that may be found in the juice. In order to lose weight, you need to consume less calories than you burn off via physical activity and alter your diet such that you have a calorie deficit[13].

Let's discuss how exactly can drinking Noni juice aid in the process of losing weight.

Noni juice contains antioxidants

Antioxidants lower the levels of inflammation, insulin resistance, and tissue fibrosis that are linked with obesity. Antioxidants have been shown over and again to be associated with weight reduction. This is likely due to the fact that antioxidants have been shown to increase the body's metabolism, particularly during exercise, which in turn may assist with weight loss.

Noni juice serves as an appetite suppressor

Studies have shown that drinking noni juice for weight loss can help reduce adipose tissue, which is another name for body fat; plasma triglyceride levels (if someone has high levels of plasma triglyceride, they will have high cholesterol, which can lead to heart strokes and high BP); and improve glucose tolerance, which can lead to a suppressed appetite and ultimately to weight loss.

Makes it easier to workout

It has also been suggested that drinking noni juice before an exercise or other physical activity will aid increase endurance. According to the findings of several studies, noni juice may be effective in warding off weariness. Antioxidants have a part in this situation as well; they assist with preventing muscle damage, and as a result, if you drink noni juice, you receive a decent quantity of antioxidants, which will aid you with your activity.

Raise your body's Ghrelin levels

Ghrelin levels are largely controlled by the amount of food consumed, and a spike in these levels may be seen either during a time of fasting or just before eating. Noni juice raises levels of the hormone ghrelin in the body, which helps the body feel full so that you don't continue consuming more food than you need to maintain your current weight (overeating decreases ghrelin levels).

Reduces fat around the abdominal organs

Visceral fat is the kind of fat that surrounds your abdominal organs and is located deep inside the body. There is a correlation between insulin resistance and visceral fat, and visceral fat may also contribute to glucose intolerance (Diabetes type two). A reduction in insulin resistance and visceral fat may be achieved with the use of noni juice for weight loss.

Lowers the level of fat and triglycerides in blood

Triglyceride levels may be lowered by drinking noni juice, as was just described. Triglycerides, often known as blood fats, are another kind of fat that may be seen circulating in the circulation alongside cholesterol.

Things to keep in mind

On the other hand, similar to other things, drinking noni juice might have certain unintended consequences. Before consuming Noni Juice, there are a few things that you really need to keep in mind.

• **Speak with your medical professional:** Before incorporating noni juice into your diet, you should speak with a medical professional to determine whether or not it is safe for you to do so. In addition, if you are taking any other medications, you should determine whether or not consuming the juice while also taking the other medicine is safe.

• **Check the dosage:** Making sure you check the dosage before consuming anything is really important. Although a few studies have shown that consuming around 750 milliliters or 25 fluid ounces of noni juice on a daily basis is not harmful, it is still best to discuss the appropriate dose with a medical professional.

- **Know if there is an underlying disease:** Despite the fact that noni juice has numerous health advantages, drinking it is not recommended for everyone. People who suffer from conditions such as chronic renal disease should not drink this. Because of this, it is highly recommended that you be checked out for any underlying problems that you could have since they might be the cause of any anomalies in your body.

Chapter 5.

How to Grow Noni

The noni plant is simple to cultivate in its natural environment, despite the widespread belief that it has mystical properties and a hefty price tag to match. Fruiting is accompanied by a range of feelings due to the unpleasant aroma of the ripe fruit, nonetheless, those who have the courage to swallow the juice extol its praises.

What you must learn about the noni fruit[12]:

• **Name:** noni plant (Morinda citrifolia).

• **Height:** 3–6m.

• **Foliage:** lustrous evergreen

• **Climate:** tropical and sub-tropical climates

• **Soil:** soil that has good drainage and has been amended with compost and manure that has had sufficient time to mature is good for its cultivation.

• **Position:** either in direct sunlight or in some shade.

• **Flowering and fruiting:** produces clusters of white, tubular flowers in the spring, followed by lumpy, creamy-colored oval-shaped fruits in the summer. Flowering and fruiting take place in the same season.

• **Feeding:** It is important not to over-fertilize since this causes plants to grow too lush and makes them more vulnerable to disease and pests. Instead, consider applying compost in the form of mulch throughout the spring.

- **Watering:** Once established, this plant is resistant to dry conditions and requires watering only when absolutely essential during lengthy periods of the dry season.

The noni fruit's outward appearance and unique qualities

The noni fruit plant may either be an evergreen shrub or tree and is rather big. The fruit is quite smelly. It is sensitive to climate, and although it is possible to grow it inside a container, the scent of the blossoms and fruit often makes this alternative less appealing.

How to start a noni fruit planting and grow it

- Plant in full sun on soil that has been amended with compost and manure and matured for some time. Because the robust root system might be a nuisance in some situations, you should avoid planting trees or shrubs too near the buildings or walkways. Because noni may grow into a tree or shrub, be sure to give the plant some room to spread out.

- After you have dug a hole that is twice as large as the pot, backfill it with some soil so that the eventual height of the plant is the same as it was when it was in the pot.

- Finish by backfilling and compacting the soil.

- Water to eliminate the voids of air that are around the roots.

- Apply mulch to prevent the growth of weeds and other competing plants.

Taking care of the noni plant

During the establishing phase, your plant will need to be watered at least twice or three times each week. After the plant has been established, it should only be watered during extended periods of drought or during hot, dry weather.

How to prune noni plant

Only prune if you wish to make the plant generally smaller, make it into a hedge, or eliminate branches that aren't needed.

Protection from diseases and insects

Insects that feed on sap, such as scale and aphids, are a potential threat to noni fruit. Sprays made of eco-oil may be used successfully to cure them, thankfully. Take the time to get rid of ants, as well, since they may lead to a rise in the number of scale insects, aphids, and sooty mold.

Propagating noni fruit trees

The noni fruit may be easily cultivated via the use of either seeds or stem cuttings. Plants that were produced from seeds are more resilient, but it takes them longer to mature.

Bringing noni fruit trees from seed to full maturity

• Take a fully ripened fruit and let it soak in water for a while.

• Transfer to a strainer and thoroughly wring out all of the pulp.

• Wash it off with water and do it again.

- After the seeds have been cleaned, spread them out on a bed of seed-raising mix and softly cover them.
- Position it over a heating pad and mist it often with water.
- When the plants have produced their first four true leaves, the seedlings may be transplanted into pots and relocated to a sheltered location that receives partial shadow. After this, the seedlings can be hardened off by gradually being moved into a position that receives full sunlight.

Root cuttings of noni fruit tree for propagation

- Take a cutting from the stem/matured branch that is about 25–30 cm long.
- Strip the lower half of the leaves by pinching your fingers over the stem and running them down the cutting.
- 3. Coat the cutting with a hormone that promotes roots or cutting, either in powder, gel, or liquid form, and then put it in a container that has been filled with propagation mix.
- 4. Maintain a consistent watering schedule and wait around three to four months before transplanting when obvious root growth has occurred.

A word of caution

Always read the label before using a product to combat weeds, diseases, or pests, and be sure to follow the directions very carefully. Additionally, make sure to wear protective gear that is appropriate for the situation. Keep any horticultural chemicals in a secure location that is inaccessible to children and animals.

Chapter 6.
Potential Side Effects of Noni Fruit

When taken internally or when an ointment containing noni is administered to the skin, noni is likely to not cause any adverse effects. On the other hand, there have been several cases of liver injury in patients who drank noni tea or juice in great quantities over an extended period of time (several weeks). It cannot be shown with absolute certainty that noni was the factor that led to these adverse outcomes. It's possible that eating dried noni fruit could make your stomach feel a little queasy.

Special precautions

Ingestion of noni should be avoided during pregnancy as well as when breastfeeding. Noni has a long history of usage in traditional medicine as an abortion-inducing agent. If you are a breastfeeding mother, it is also recommended that you stay away from noni. There is insufficient evidence to support the claim that consuming noni while breastfeeding is safe.

Noni includes a significant quantity of potassium, which might cause kidney difficulties. This could provide a challenge, particularly for those who already have a renal illness. After consuming noni juice, one individual with renal problems was reported to have had excessive amounts of potassium in their blood. If you have renal issues, you should avoid using noni.

Noni has been associated with a number of incidences of liver illness due to its consumption. If you have liver illness, you should avoid taking noni[14].

Possible interactions with other drugs

If your physician has recommended some drugs to treat your illness, your physician or pharmacist may already be aware of any potential drug interactions or adverse effects, and they may be keeping an eye on you to ensure that you do not experience any of them. Do not begin, stop, or modify the dose of that drug or any other medicine until first getting more information from your physician, other healthcare practitioners, or pharmacist[15].

Medication for conditions related to high blood pressure (ACE inhibitors)

• Rating for Interaction: Moderately Effective

Take care while putting these things together. Have a conversation with your primary care physician. Taking some drugs to treat high blood pressure might cause an increase in the amount of potassium found in the blood. If you take these drugs for high blood pressure and consume noni juice at the same time, it is possible that your blood potassium level may become excessively high. Captopril (Capoten), enalapril (Vasotec), lisinopril (Prinivil, Zestril), and ramipril (Altace) are just a few of the drugs that are used to treat high blood pressure. There are many more.

Angiotensin receptor blockers, sometimes known as ARBs

- Rating for Interaction: Moderately Effective

Take care while putting these things together. Have a conversation with your primary care physician. A potentially dangerously high level of potassium in the blood might be the result of consuming noni juice in conjunction with some hypertension drugs.

Candesartan (Atacand), irbesartan (Avapro), telmisartan (Micardis), eprosartan (Teveten), and losartan (Cozaar) are just a few of the drugs that are available to treat high blood pressure. Other options include eprosartan (Teveten) and telmisartan (Micardis).

Medication for conditions related to low blood pressure (Antihypertensive drugs)

- Rating for Interaction: Moderately Effective

Take care while putting these things together. Have a conversation with your primary care physician. Some individuals find that consuming noni juice brings their blood pressure down. If you take drugs to bring your blood pressure down and noni at the same time, you run the risk of having your blood pressure drop to an unsafe level. However, it is unknown if this is a major cause for worry. If you are already taking medicine for blood pressure-related problems, you should limit the amount of noni juice you consume.

Captopril (Capoten), Enalapril (Vasotec), Losartan (Cozaar), Valsartan (Diovan), Diltiazem (Cardizem), Amlodipine (Norvasc), Hydrochlorothiazide (HydroDiuril), Furosemide (Lasix) etc.

Medications that have the potential to cause liver damage (Hepatotoxic drugs)

- Rating for Interaction: Moderately Effective

It is possible to enhance the risk of liver damage by using noni in conjunction with medicine that might possibly be harmful to the liver. If you are currently taking a drug that is dangerous to the liver, you should not consume noni.

A number of drugs, including acetaminophen (Tylenol and other brands), amiodarone (Cordarone), carbamazepine (Tegretol), isoniazid (INH), methotrexate (Rheumatrex), methyldopa (Aldomet), fluconazole (Diflucan), itraconazole (Sporanox), erythromycin (Erythrocin), etc.

Blood thinning medicines (Warfarin)

- Rating for Interaction: Moderately Effective

Take care while putting these things together. Have a conversation with your primary care physician. Warfarin, also known as Coumadin, is used to reduce the rate at which blood clots. It is possible that drinking noni juice can lessen the effectiveness of the anticoagulant drug warfarin (Coumadin). The likelihood of a blood clot forming is increased as a result of this.

Water pills (Potassium-sparing diuretics)

- Rating for Interaction: Moderately Effective

Take care while putting these things together. Have a conversation with your primary care physician.

The noni fruit has a rather high potassium content. A number of different "water tablets" have been shown to raise potassium levels in the body. When used with noni, some "water tablets" may cause an unsafely high level of potassium to build up in the body.

Amiloride (trade name: Midamor), spironolactone (trade name: Aldactone), and triamterene (Dyrenium) are all examples of "water pills" that raise potassium levels in the body.

Dosage

The optimal dosage of noni is determined by a number of factors, including the age of the user, their current state of health, and a number of other situations. There is not a sufficient amount of scientific knowledge available at this time to identify a suitable range of dosages for noni. It is vital to keep in mind that natural products are not always guaranteed to be safe and that doses may sometimes be quite significant. Before using, ensure that you have read and understood all applicable instructions found on product labels, and check in with your pharmacist, your doctor, or another qualified healthcare expert.

Safety

There is a lack of consensus on the safety of noni juice due to the limited number of human research that has been conducted to investigate its dosage and potential adverse effects. For instance, the results of a short research conducted on healthy people suggested that it is safe to consume noni juice on a daily basis in amounts of up to 25 ounces (750 ml). On the other hand, in 2005 there were a few reports of people ingesting noni juice who ended up having liver damage. The European Food Safety Authority (EFSA) subsequently reassessed the fruit and came to the conclusion that the effects were not caused by noni juice on its own.

In 2009, the European Food Safety Authority (EFSA) published a further statement indicating that noni juice is safe for consumption by the general public. However, specialists from EFSA did note that certain people may have a greater susceptibility to the harmful consequences of liver damage than others. Noni juice should also be avoided by those who have chronic renal disease or kidney issues because of its high potassium content, which may cause dangerously high levels of this component in the blood. In addition, noni juice may have an effect on the way some drugs work as discussed above, so it's essential to discuss the use of noni juice with your primary care physician before beginning[16].

Have a lot of sugar

Because there are a lot of variations between brands of noni juice, some of them may have a lot of sugar in them. In addition to this, it is often combined with other fruit liquids that are very sweet in taste. In fact, there are around 8 grams of sugar in 3.5 ounces (100 milliliters) of noni juice. According to a number of studies, consuming sugar-sweetened drinks like noni juice may put you at a greater risk for developing metabolic disorders such as nonalcoholic fatty liver disease (NAFLD) and type II diabetes. Therefore, it is probably preferable to drink noni juice in moderation or to avoid it altogether, if you restrict the amount of sugar you consume in your diet.

Warnings

The following are some of the most common adverse reactions to noni juice:

- Diarrhea (which has a laxative effect)
- Acute hepatitis
- Liver toxicity
- Hyperkalemia

If you have an allergy to noni juice or any of the substances present in it, you should not use beach mulberry, great morinda, Indian mulberry, mengkudu, Morinda citrifolia, noni, nono, nonu, or Tahitian noni. Make sure that youngsters can't get their hands on it. In the event of an overdose, seek emergency medical attention or make contact with a poison control center.

Concomitant use with powerful CYP3A4 inducers (such as rifampin, rifabutin, phenobarbital, phenytoin, carbamazepine, and St. John's wort) considerably lowers the effectiveness of noni juice. Immediate release preparations should be made (either sublingually or orally) for urgent or emergent hypertension in case of overdosage.

Pregnancy and Nursing: There is currently no information available on the safety of consuming noni juice either during pregnancy or while breastfeeding. Consult your doctor.

Conclusion

Noni has a very high concentration of vitamin C and may provide anti-inflammatory advantages, including the reduction of pain as well as improvements in immunological health and the ability to exercise for longer periods of time. It is important to remember that commercial cultivars are sometimes combined with other juices and might have a high amount of sugar. Evidence gained from human research overwhelmingly suggests that noni juice has a higher level of antioxidant activity than other fruits. Because of this activity as well as its interaction with the immune system and inflammatory pathways, noni juice may be responsible for a significant portion of the health benefits that have been documented. These health benefits may include protection against the toxicities caused by tobacco smoke (such as the protection of DNA, normalization of blood lipids, control of systemic inflammation, and reduction of homocysteine), improvement of joint pain and mobility, increased physical endurance, increased immune activity, weight management, maintenance of bone health in women, control of blood pressure, and improvement of gum health.

This is something that must be kept in mind, as it is very essential. The use of noni juice is probably risk-free. However, if you are on certain drugs or if you have renal issues, you may want to check with your medical provider before consuming this. The data that is now available does have a few broad restrictions that prevent it from being completely applicable to noni juice products. Commercial noni juice products have varying phytochemical and nutritional profiles due to a combination of geographical characteristics and post-growth factors (harvesting, storage, shipping, processing, and formulation). Variations in biological activity are probably going to be a direct consequence of differences in phytochemical profiles.

References

1. Wang, M.-Y., et al., *Morinda citrifolia (Noni): a literature review and recent advances in Noni research.* Acta Pharmacologica Sinica, 2002. **23**(12): p. 1127-1141.

2. Chan-Blanco, Y., et al., *The noni fruit (Morinda citrifolia L.): A review of agricultural research, nutritional and therapeutic properties.* Journal of Food Composition and Analysis, 2006. **19**(6): p. 645-654.

3. Abou Assi, R., et al., *Morinda citrifolia (Noni): A comprehensive review on its industrial uses, pharmacological activities, and clinical trials.* Arabian Journal of Chemistry, 2017. **10**(5): p. 691-707.

4. West, B.J., et al., *The Potential Health Benefits of Noni Juice: A Review of Human Intervention Studies.* Foods, 2018. **7**(4).

5. Wang, M.Y., et al., *Morinda citrifolia (Noni): a literature review and recent advances in Noni research.* Acta Pharmacol Sin, 2002. **23**(12): p. 1127-41.

6. Nelson, S.C., *Noni cultivation in Hawaii.* 2001.

7. Ali, M., M. Kenganora, and S.N. Manjula, *Health benefits of Morinda citrifolia (Noni): A review.* Pharmacognosy Journal, 2016. **8**(4).

8. Bhatia, R., K. Thapliyal, and D. Kumar, *Phytochemical and Therapeutic Aspects of Morinda citrifolia L.(Noni Plant): A Review.* Research Journal of Pharmacognosy and Phytochemistry, 2015. **7**(3): p. 167-174.

9. West, B.J., C.J. Jensen, and J. Westendorf, *Noni juice is not hepatotoxic.* World Journal of Gastroenterology: WJG, 2006. **12**(22): p. 3616.

10. Basar, S., et al., *Analgesic and antiinflammatory activity of Morinda citrifolia L.(Noni) fruit.* Phytotherapy Research: An International Journal Devoted to Pharmacological and Toxicological Evaluation of Natural Product Derivatives, 2010. **24**(1): p. 38-42.

11. Gupta, R.K. and A.K. Patel, *Do the health claims made for Morinda citrifolia (Noni) harmonize with current scientific knowledge and evaluation of its biological effects.* Asian Pacific Journal of Cancer Prevention, 2013. **14**(8): p. 4495-4499.

12. Nelson, S.C. and C.R. Elevitch, *Noni: the complete guide for consumers and growers.* 2006: PAR.

13. West, B.J., et al., *The potential health benefits of noni juice: a review of human intervention studies.* Foods, 2018. **7**(4): p. 58.

14. Sharma, Y., et al., *Noni: a new medicinal plant for the tropics.* African journal of plant science, 2014. **8**(5): p. 243-247.

15. Almeida, É.S., D. de Oliveira, and D. Hotza, *Properties and applications of Morinda citrifolia (noni): A review.* Comprehensive Reviews in Food Science and Food Safety, 2019. **18**(4): p. 883-909.

16. Mueller, B.A., et al., *Noni juice (Morinda citrifolia): hidden potential for hyperkalemia?*

American Journal of Kidney Diseases, 2000. **35**(2): p. 310-312.